CONTENTS

Copyright 2019 © by Juliano Statdlober.

The author of this work is the copyright owner.

This book is a result of an independent production, written, edited, and published by the author to contribute to the dissemination of information on prostate cancer. Reports of personal experience are presented.

The author is not a Medical Doctor. Do not use any content of this book as a basis for any decision on diagnosis or treatment.

Always consult a Medical Doctor.

The text was not submitted to a formal language review process to make the book more affordable. Some complacency is expected for any semantic, spelling, or grammar mistakes.

The reproduction of the entire content or parts of it is strictly prohibited without previous authorization from the author.

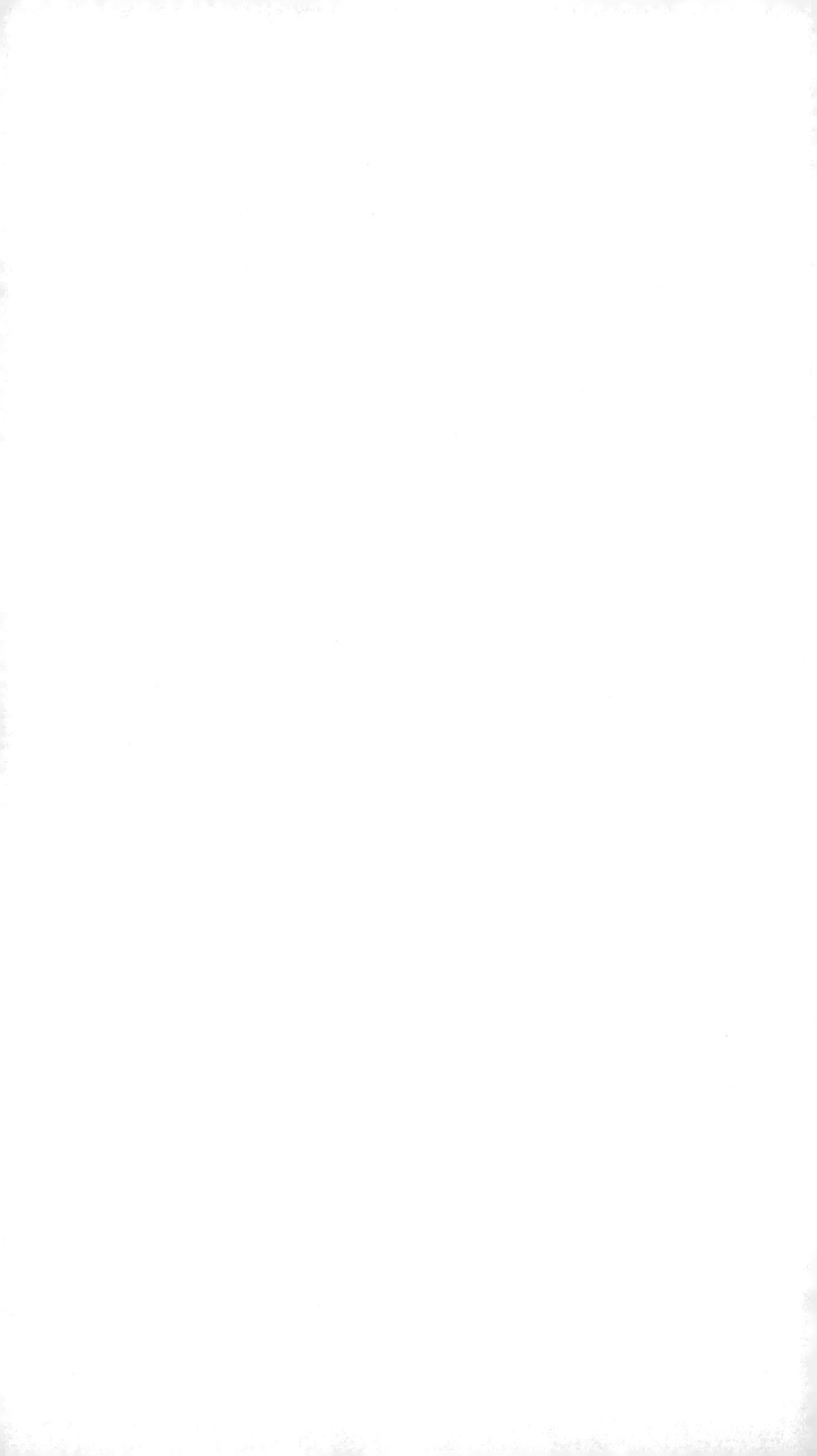

ABOUT THE BOOK

This book portrays the perspective of a prostate cancer patient to other patients, their families, and acquaintances. It is not a medical or scientific text, and it is plain and easy to understand.

Prostate cancer is the most common among men, right after skin cancer.

It is essential that everyone, after a certain age, perform periodic examinations to ensure that, in case a prostate cancer is detected, it is as early as possible.

- Why?
- What is the prostate, and what is its function?
- What happens to a man without a prostate?
- How does the diagnosis of cancer work?

> What are its steps?
- If the cancer is confirmed, how is the treatment process?
- What are the emotions that arise? What are the fears?
- What are the possible consequences?
- What are the treatments? How does prostatectomy work?

All these answers and some others are in this book with the view of a patient of prostate cancer. It explains the journey from the investigation, through diagnosis, treatment, and healing. Some suggestions are presented by the author, resulting from his learning about the whole process.

For whom can this book be useful?

- For all who seek better information about prostate cancer, the importance of its early diagnosis, and its treatment.
- For those who are diagnosed with prostate cancer, finding information and some critical answers, to which I, the author, would like to have had access to when I discovered that I had cancer.
- For relatives and friends of a patient, who can understand the feelings that can arise with the disease, to deal better with the situation.

A LIVED, FELT AND SHARED STORY

I have to confess, it wasn't an easy decision. I admit that I have always had, and still have, an absolute embarrassment about sharing feelings and emotions.

Until I was faced with a threatening situation of diagnosis of prostate cancer.

I will report in the book my personal journey. For now, I think it is important to note that I decided to write, first of all, to try to "help myself." It was a way to deal with the bunch of frightening, omnipresent and oppressive thoughts, from the first suspicion, through the confirmation of the diagnosis, to the final outcome.

I will start with some information about the prostate and its function, and then highlight the importance of early diagnosis of prostate cancer.

Several topics will deal with thoughts and feelings that arose when I came across the reality of having cancer, such as fear, hope, and denial.

In one chapter, I will address the question of talking about it (or not) with the people around, such as my family, for example.

I will also describe in more detail how the diagnosis and treatment of prostate cancer works.

I ended up finding in the written text a way to "speak" freely to myself, without censorship and without harassing or scaring anyone, in a legitimate monologue.

I did an experiment, and I ended up realizing that writing helped me to relieve the anguish, certainly by becoming a practice that was transmuted into a kind of personal catharsis. Popularly it is said that it is important to "put things out."

I started to experiment with writing as therapy. Then I realized that it became a useful tool for dealing with anxiety peaks. Later I will address the curious impossibility of not thinking about something, which makes it difficult to control anxiety.

No less important is to mention that most contents are the result of records and notes made as the timeline of the ritual and the marathon unfolded. I will also explain the rites of the diagnosis and the marathon of the treatment. The thoughts and their anguish, related to each stage, were more real that way. I came to the conclusion that I could not be faithful to the feeling if I wrote everything later, as for example, after being healed.

Several notes were made when I was anxiously awaiting the diagnosis, others later when I had the confirmation of having cancer, but before performing a radical prostatectomy surgery. Rereading those records, I can relive the feelings more clearly to try to report them in the most authentic way possible. I can remember how I lived a mixture of thoughts tempered by fear and hope as if each one of the spices took turns and prevailed at its time.

In short, my first reason for writing, therefore, was self-help for myself, with the forgiveness of redundancy.

Another reason that encouraged me to write is that I believe it can help to clarify about the disease and how the diagnosis and treatment work. All from one personal point of view of a patient.

Countless content on the Internet about prostate cancer is available, but most of it is technical or written by doctors. What I've been willing to report offers a different perspective than the one that results from Googling about cancer and reading medical or scientific articles.

Interestingly, in comparative terms, it seems to me that there is much more dissemination of information, clarification, and support for breast cancer patients. Of course, they are different diseases, with varying impacts and treatments. Still, I believe that men also have the right to have access to more knowledge about their prevalent type of cancer.

I'm going to deal with how things work because I've been through them in an experience I've had. I intend to share, in addition to information, thoughts, and feelings. I would like to have had access to this if it had been written by others before when I started dealing with this situation.

It would be great to know if more people felt what I felt and how they handled a similar circumstance. In other words, I would very much like to have had more information before, but I had no one to ask.

I know this might have scared me more, but who knows, it might have reassured me?

Maybe I could have helped myself to fantasize less...

I believe I could have worked as a kind of virtual support group.

If it would have been good for me, who knows if it would have been suitable for other people?

MEET THE PROSTATE

I knew little and was not interested in the function of the prostate in the body unless I thought that maybe it only existed to get cancer.

I reproduce below some information that I learned, for leveling of knowledge. I believe that no matter how basic they may be for many, they may be useful for many other people.

Briefly, without scientific deepening, the prostate is a gland that is part of the male genital system, whose function is to produce a liquid that surrounds and protects the spermatozoa and is part of the semen.

It is located below the bladder, in front of the rectum, involving the urethra. The urethra is a channel that connects the bladder to the penis. The urethra, therefore, passes through the prostate. This explains why an enlarged prostate (which is called hyperplasia) or one affected by a tumor can make urination difficult, precisely because it compresses the urethra.

The seminal fluid is produced in another organ, the seminal vesicles. The semen is formed with what is provided in the prostate and contains the spermatozoa generated in the testicles. A man can live, therefore, ordinarily without his prostate but does not ejaculate semen anymore.

A last vital element to be mentioned is related to erection. Some nerves pass near or along the prostate, responsible for the stimuli that are necessary for an erection.

Some relevant information, for which I have heard doubts:

It is important to stress out that the removal of the prostate does not end with the sexual life. Erectile dysfunction can be caused by possible sequelae resulting from the surgery of treatment of cancer, described in the sequence.

The fact that a man does not ejaculate does not characterize him as impotent since impotence is the inability to have an erection. An erection obviously can happen without ejaculation. All men who remove the prostate and seminal vesicles become sterile, which means they can no longer bear children.

Being sterile also does not mean being impotent,

they are different things.

Prostate cancer and its treatment can lead to two consequences, difficulty in controlling urination and sexual impotence (AKA erectile dysfunction).

The first, because the surgical removal of the prostate causes the urethra to be disconnected from the bladder, with subsequent reconnection, which can leave some deficiency in sphincter control. The sphincter is a kind of valve that opens or closes to let urine out of the bladder. Moreover, depending on the location, the urethra and the sphincter itself may be directly affected by the tumor. Even without surgical intervention, urinary incontinence can result from radiotherapy, which in turn can also impact the urethra and bladder.

As for the impact on erection, the damage can occur by contact or harm to the nerves responsible for sexual stimulation, especially when they are close to the prostate. These nerves can be affected by surgical intervention and radiotherapy, as well as in some cases by the tumor itself.

THE IMPORTANCE OF EARLY DIAGNOSIS OF PROSTATE CANCER

I'll start by writing about a fact that may seem curious to many, surprise or even cause strangeness:

Prostate cancer is a severe disease.

There is a lot of misinformation about this disease.

Some may even think that it is not so severe because a lot is said nowadays that the probability of cure is very high. Perhaps there is also a myth that prostate cancer is something unimportant and almost a common disease.

Know, dear reader, that reality is different. According to zerocancer.org, every 17 minutes, another American man dies from prostate cancer. That's a little more than 86 deaths per day and 31,620 this year, enough to fill an entire baseball stadium.

It is essential, therefore, that the diagnosis is made as soon as possible.

And why diagnose soon?

Because prostate cancer is considered a malignant tumor, containing cells that can "invade" other parts of the body, causing so-called metastasis. That's where the big problem lies.

Prostate cancer can cause metastasis in bones and lymph nodes. It can invade the rectum, bladder, ureters, and lungs, causing much suffering, compromise in quality of life, and a high possibility of death.

Important note by the author: As I mentioned earlier, I am not a doctor, but this information is abundantly available in the medical literature.

If a metastasis occurs, it changes all. It is popularly said that "a prostate cancer detected, in the beginning, has a high chance of cure." What it actually means is that it is better to fight it and heal it before it goes beyond the perimeter of the prostate.

The obvious conclusion, therefore, is that if someone has prostate cancer, it should be diagnosed as soon as possible, "at the beginning," before it spreads to other tissues or organs.

To prevent and ensure that the diagnosis is made as soon as possible, it is necessary to consult a urologist regularly, there is no other way.

There is, therefore, a big mistake to avoid.

Men who do not regularly follow up on their diagnosis, thinking that they do not need to do so if they do not feel anything.

This is a mistake that can be very expensive.

Many manifestations of prostate cancer are totally asymptomatic, that is, they are not felt, as in my case. I didn't feel anything different at all, be it pain, burning, bleeding, or even difficulty to urinate. This seems to me to be another myth that one should only consult a urologist if there is a change in urination.

There is no "right" age to start visiting a doctor regularly. Many speak in 50 years. Still, I suggest that from the age of 40, all men should have regular consultations - fortunately, that is what I did, which certainly helped in my early diagnosis and cure.

How investigation works

I think it is appropriate to clarify how prostate cancer investigation works (in the medical literature, the diagnosis is sometimes called screening).

The process begins with a blood test ordered by the doctor to evaluate the level of PSA, the result of which indicates the antigens produced by the prostate. There is no standard reference for a "good" level of PSA detected under examination. This is because it is taken into account along with other factors, including patient age, genetic predisposition, general health condition, as well as other criteria resulting from a clinical analysis by the urologist.

For most men, it is enough to repeat this routine annually, a consultation, and a blood test. By the way, it is little effort to think about health, isn't it?

Over time, I learned a few things about diagnosing prostate cancer that made me confused and insecure. High PSA may indicate cancer, but there is no official standard for what is high. The fact that a certain level of PSA is considered high does not necessarily imply that there is cancer. The variance can be caused by prostatitis, prostate infection, for example. On the other hand, to further complicate matters, having low PSA does not mean a guarantee that you do not have cancer!

Depending on the results of the PSA test and other

factors, the doctor may decide to have a rectal examination, which consists of touching the prostate through the rectum. It is done for checking the size of the prostate, and possible changes in its consistency.

Here's a fact: there is an absurd prejudice among some (or many) men against the defamed rectal examination.

It surprises me that in the 21st century, many men fear this exam or feel embarrassed about it. For those who consider masculinity "threatened" by the invasion, it is essential to clarify that this will not happen in all consultations. It is possible to maintain good diagnostic security without going through the procedure, leaving only the consultation and the blood test.

Let's face it, if and when someone has to undergo a touch test, what is the problem?

CANCER, ONE OF THE GREAT FEARS OF THE COLLECTIVE UNCONSCIOUS

I can't say for sure if the fear is really collective or if it's personal. Still, I believe that cancer haunts most people, if not the vast majority. Many don't even like to speak the word - some people refer to it as "Big C."

All my life, from a very young age, I have been haunted by cancer. I lost my mother to cancer when I was 18, which, by the way, is not irrelevant in anyone's life. My father had prostate cancer, and my grandfather died from prostate cancer. My grandmother had breast cancer, and I still had a cousin who passed away very young due to cancer.

All right, if you analyze the context and think about it, maybe it's a dread that's more mine than collective, the result of personal experiences. Since I was very young, I have heard conversations that the great challenge of science is to find a cure for cancer. It was (or still is) an incurable disease that brings a lot of suffering.

Among the negative highlights given by the media and social networks is terrible news about public people who have cancer. I consider myself a very empathetic person, and this news really causes me discomfort. I keep thinking about how those who discover such a diagnosis would feel, that is, how terrible it is to have cancer.

THE RITUAL OF PROSTATE CANCER DIAGNOSIS

As I have already written, the cancer ghost has been part of my life, haunting me for a long time. Many times it has played the role of supporting actor, along with everything else that involves living, such as routine, work, family, joys, sorrows, disappointments, and happiness. Despite not being the lead actor, he was always there, bothering me.

One day my father was diagnosed with prostate cancer. I started visiting a urologist regularly since I was 40 years old when I discovered that I became a case of attention, due to a possible genetic predisposition.

In one of the annual reviews, at the time at the age of 40 and a few, I had a first unexpected PSA level result. I remember until today, it was 1.6. At the time, with everything else being within normality (including the rectal touch examination), I became a case of even more attention.

It is important to register that the genetic predisposition may or may not result in cancer, and there are many cases of non-occurrence in descendants. If your father or grandfather has had it, it does not necessarily mean that you will have it. If you have an ascendant with prostate cancer, do not hesitate to consult a urologist from the age of 40.

Some years passed with the routine of annual reviews, when, at 50 years of age, I had a first more significant increase in the level of PSA. At the time, it rose to just over 4 (the levels had been varying slowly, from 1.6 to 2.6).

For the first time, I felt a more real than phantasmagoric fear of the possibility of a cancer diagnosis. I went through what I call a diagnostic ritual, which resulted in a happy outcome of the absence of neoplasia.

Three years later, the ritual started again after a PSA result of 6.7, when then the investigation ended with an undesired outcome: carcinoma, that is, cancer.

Things as bad as this, a diagnosis of cancer, were

always other people's misfortune, until one day it sounded an alarm, the floor opened and the person diagnosed was me.

I even thought that this paragraph was unnecessary, an excess of redundancy, but I decided to write it down. It's about emphasizing once again the importance of the periodic, annual visit to the urologist. As obvious as it may seem, as natural as it sounds, and as inconceivable as it may be to me, we hear a lot that many men from the age of 50 do not visit a urologist regularly.

Unbelievable!

It is essential to register (once again) that even with the confirmed diagnosis, I felt absolutely nothing different, no physical symptoms. Some men think that they should only look for a urologist if something is abnormal, such as, for example, feeling some burning or difficult to urinate. It is absolute nonsense. It is not true.

Back to the diagnostic ritual, my goal in describing this process, with its stages, is to clarify and explain how prostate cancer investigation works. I am not a doctor, and what I write in this chapter has no scientific authentication or basis, is based on what I have learned from my personal experience, that is no longer so small.

In consultation, the doctor requests a PSA test (a blood test;) depending on the result, and according to his criteria, he can perform the (absurdly feared) rectal touch test. Perhaps because of the macho culture, some men fear this test as if it were a threat to their masculinity. Comfortable is not, but in certain situations, it is essential.

Some indicators evaluated jointly by the doctor lead to a possible deepening of the diagnosis, such as age, genetic predisposition, PSA level, and evaluation of the rectal touch test. The sequence of investigation is made with several steps if any suspicion arises.

It was the ritual that I followed every time, and I believe, therefore, that it is the standard for all cases. As I have already mentioned, I speak of personal experiences, this text is not a medical essence, and there may be urologists who proceed differently.

The first examination is an ultrasound of the abdomen and bladder, for which, I understand, one of the main objectives is to check the size of the prostate, some possible more prominent abnormality, and the urine residue that remains in the bladder after urinating. It's a relatively quick exam, and waiting for the diagnosis has never caused me much discomfort or impatience. I always did this procedure annually in a general check-up, so it was something routine for me.

After that, I had a new appointment with the doctor. On this latest visit, he requested an MRI of the prostate. I had done an MRI before, due to some investigation related to a running injury if I'm not mistaken.

Many people complain of claustrophobia through the "tube" of the MRI, but this had not bothered me. The first time I had to do a prostate resonance, I remember thinking, "I don't know why the other times it wasn't asked for, just to eliminate any doubt."

I scheduled the exam, arrived on the spot, followed the procedure of waiting for the registration, made the registration, waited for it, tic, tac, tic tac. When my turn came, I changed clothes. Wearing that laboratory apron, out of curiosity, I asked the assistant:

"How long does it take?"

I asked, thinking about something from work if there would be time to be back at the office in 45 minutes or an hour (it was what was going through my head).

When the answer came:

"This resonance is one of the most time-consuming. It takes between 40 and 50 minutes."

It took me a while to assimilate. I even thought I heard it wrong. I asked for confirmation. That was it. I was never claustrophobic; when I had an MRI of another kind before, it was a 10 to 15-minute thing; I don't remember having any bad feelings.

This time, however, those 40 minutes impacted me. I remember as if it were today the sensation that I started to feel when the stretcher was sliding into the "tube."

Just before I came in, I had another "surprise" when I figured out that I couldn't move my legs or move my abdomen at all, or I would have to start all over again. I shouldn't even think of coughing.

The sensation of entering the "tube" to stay for 40 or 50 minutes, already with the desire to move the legs from the beginning, is not something comfortable to face. It may seem exaggerated, even fresh, so I propose that you, reader, lie down now and stay 5 minutes without moving your legs, resting still. Is it easy?

The thought that began to cross my mind as soon as the exam started, with that turbine noise and beats mixed with an electric buzzing sound, was, "how long has it been?" I tried to start counting the seconds, not knowing if my count was fast or slow. When I got there by 200, it would mean that it would have been 3 minutes and little. Or was it much less? How much longer would it be? Along it comes an almost uncontrollable urge to move your legs. How nice it would be to bend your knees! I have to think of something else.

I look up, there's a tube inches from my eyes, which seems to be getting smaller. I was trying to fill my lungs with air, and it didn't seem to work.

That was my first prostate resonance right after the first "jump" to the PSA level. I was very anxious about the result, but still, during the exam, I thought more than once about ringing the bell and asking to stop. *"Tough luck, I won't be able to take it to the end, I'll get out of here and see what I can do,"* I thought the most. I think it was the longest 48 minutes of my life (it was the time it took, they told me when I asked later).

Then came the next step of the ritual, to wait for the result, that is, the report of the resonance. As I was always impressed and amazed by the subject, and once that was the first time, the waiting was very uncomfortable, making me very impatient. The report with results would be sent by e-mail, and two days before the promised deadline, it became very tense to look at the mailbox, waiting for it (wait for results, let's say, turned out to be kind of routine for me).

On the day that the sender appeared in the inbox, I remember well the sensation, increased heartbeat, and heavier breathing, in a perfect classic manifestation of anxiety.

This first report said something like there was a suggestion of signs of changes in cells and tissues, which were not identifiable. It indicated, therefore, that there could be something, but it was not possible to confirm it.

As this raised a strong suspicion, there should be a more in-depth investigation, so the next examination indicated by the doctor was a biopsy.

To clarify how things work, here is a prostate biopsy: it is a transrectal examination performed with the aid of ultrasonography, whose objective is, literally, the removal of pieces of the prostate for pathological analysis of tissue samples.

The objective of a biopsy is to verify if there are differentiated cells, that is, different from healthy prostate cells - suggesting cancer. There are about 15 pieces collected, a little less, a little more.

The exam itself does not cause significant discomfort when performed with sedation, which, for us, laymen, has the same effect of general anesthesia.

The preparation is relatively simple; you take an antibiotic from the day before and for a few days afterward, besides fasting for 8 hours before the exam. And that's it. At the time of the examination, general blackout, and when one opens the eyes, it passed. No pain, no discomfort.

Except when, at the time of the second biopsy, due to one more PSA elevation and a more significant suspicion detected in a new MRI (but not yet conclusive), I had decided to seek another opinion, changing doctors, following a recommendation of an acquaintance. The procedure suggested by this doctor, however, left me somewhat traumatized.

According to him, who is a highly respected urologist, the ideal would be to do the biopsy in a laboratory where the ultrasound equipment was better, with sharper images, which would increase the probability of finding some alteration visually to make the tissue collection at the right points. In other words, there would be a higher chance of finding the positions indicated by resonance imaging.

Only that, as the biopsy would be in the laboratory, there was no hospital structure. Therefore, there would be no anesthesiologist available. In other words, there would not be sedation for the biopsy.

It was my choice. I could choose to do it in a hospital, as on the previous occasion. In the doctor's opinion, however, the visualization of the ultrasound would be better at the place where he suggested it. It might have been for this reason that nothing was wrong in the first biopsy.

What is a layman does at this time, anxious for a more accurate biopsy? He accepts the suggestion. I did.

If the resonance was painful, readers could try to imagine a biopsy without sedation, with the patient awake and no anesthesia. I confess that it is too embarrassing to describe the test in detail. Still, the feeling of being conscious and sensing when pieces are extracted, with equipment that cuts with impact, is indescribable.

I have heard from women and read that the breast biopsy is similar because it takes place in a laboratory, without sedation. I can't, and I don't intend to compare, maybe it's also something close to a medieval torture session.

After this examination, there was a new (impatient) waiting for the result. Impacted by the increase in PSA and by the more forceful suggestion of resonance that something might be wrong, the wait for the biopsy report was even tenser. I remember very well the day the e-mail arrived with the result. I was in the gym doing weight training.

When I saw the message, sitting on a piece of equipment, I clearly remember when I was opening the PDF, the anxiety was stronger than the first time. I wear reading glasses, but obviously, I didn't have them at the gym. It is tough to read on the cell phone, even more so without glasses, the letters are all scrambled, I had to zoom in on the screen to find the words so desired: "***Absence of neoplasm.***" I clearly remember that I stood up and realized that I was dizzy; there is no way to describe the sensation. It was one of the best I can remember all my life, knowing that I didn't have cancer.

In the meantime, between the resonance and the final report of the biopsy, I remember that I felt a lot of emotional impacts, to the point of not doing some things for absolute lack of motivation, feeling a certain prostration for the activities of the day-by-day. If I look at my GPS running statistics today, I see a break when I didn't run for a couple of months during that period, which confirms that not even one of the things I like the most was what I wanted to do.

Returning to the doctor with the biopsy report,

very happy, I received a very detailed explanation, which left me discouraged. I have been learning many things along my journey, and some of these lessons have not always been pleasant.

In short, I learned that:

> The fact that a biopsy gives a negative result does not mean that there is not something wrong; it just means that it didn't found something. It just means that the samples collected have no cancer cells.

The fact that the samples are free of cancer cells can be casual since, in some situations, it is challenging that the collection is made precisely in the region indicated by the resonance. In cases where cancer is not throughout all the prostate, this situation can happen.

To put it bluntly, these are somewhat random possibilities. Of course, there is an optimistic point in a negative diagnosis, since cancer is not all over the prostate. It does not mean, however, that you do not have the disease.

Shit!

I didn't get rid of the ghosts, not even with a negative biopsy. The conclusion is that I would have to continue monitoring PSA. Also, if it were relatively high, if the level did not vary, there would be no cause for concern. It was a matter of doing this every six months and maintaining the annual consultation routine.

And so it was, I continued to take PSA exams every six months. Stable levels, with one of the tests, even reduced, actually a small reduction, but after all, it was a reduction.

What a good thing. It was two years when the ghosts had become comrades ghosts, and I had almost forgotten them.

After the experience with the last doctor, I decided to change again.

I searched for new opinions and indications from acquaintances and marked a new revision with a new professional. A new cycle was about to start, with a new PSA exam. Intimately I was convinced that, due to the last measured reduction, it was a ritual that would end at the beginning, since the touch examination did not indicate any alteration (in this case, given the history, the doctor did the touch examination already in the first consultation).

The result of this last PSA test was unexpected. From 4.2 about six months earlier, the level had risen to 6.7. Something unforeseen and suspicious was happening. I learned of this result on July 23, 2019, when my journey started.

After exposing my past trauma from the biopsy, my

new doctor reassured me: "you don't usually do any more biopsy without sedation." He recommended resonance imaging at an institution that had a technology that would allow, if necessary, the use of ultrasound fusion images in a subsequent biopsy, which would be more accurate. It was an analogy to using the resonance images as a GPS map to navigate and guide the biopsy.

For this new resonance, I relied on the help of a professional to treat the anxiety, and, on his recommendation, I prepared myself with an anxiolytic; I must confess that the experience was much more acceptable. The anticipation was worse than the exam. The MRI itself may have been less painful, but I cannot say the same for the result.

After waiting again for the report with a good dose of anxiety and impatience, distressing due to the result of high PSA came the results report, this time with an indication of a high probability of neoplasia (cancer), given a diagnosis represented by an acronym of **PI RADS-4**.

Without going into technical-scientific details, which I do not master, a PI-RADS is an international score that goes from 1 to 5. One represents a very low probability and five very high probability of cell differentiation, or in other words, of having cancer.

A PIRADS-4 means "clinically significant cancer is

likely.

To me, this result sounded deterministic. Although I tried to cling to a chance of not having cancer (it was not yet clinically a confirmation, as it depended on a new biopsy), I began to prepare myself to accept that I was likely to have it. As incredible as it may seem, the doubt was perhaps as distressing as the possibility of confirmation.

A high possibility was not yet a proven diagnosis, but the mental impact was burdensome. As I began to prepare for fatality, a voice of stunted and dehydrated hope was still trying to tell me that it might be nothing.

When I realized, I was fantasizing about opening the e-mail of the report and reading the "absence of neoplasm," thinking about repeating the sensation already experienced before. How good it will be, I thought. Then came another stronger thought, like the typical cliché of the little devil speaking in the other ear: "but how is it going to be nothing with this result of resonance? Of course, there is something.

> It's incredible how the human unconscious (or at least mine) can't cope well with any threat to well-being or life. What the archetype of cancer represents is a reminder of the infallibility of death.

No matter how much one tries to rationalize about

the advances in medicine, about the probabilities of healing prostate cancer when detected in the beginning, the unconscious is master at disturbing when disturbed. Strange as it may seem, I was not afraid of dying, only of having cancer.

If any positive fact happened in this new cycle of the ritual, is that the e-mail with the report arrived unexpectedly days before the prediction. I wasn't even expecting it, when on a Monday morning, at work, the result appeared on the screen, among other day-to-day e-mails. It even took me a while to realize what it was, so unexpected that it was the arrival. Unexpected was also my reaction, almost automatic.

I don't know-how, or maybe because I "already knew," I immediately opened the PDF without hesitating, and on the larger computer screen, it was easier to find the result in the final part. Soon I saw the words "carcinoma" and "neoplasm." Immediately, knowing without wanting to accept, I went to the browser and googled the words.

It was then that I felt a sensation never experienced before in my life, as opposed to the one when I had read a result that said I had no cancer. Now I knew I did.

I remember well that the google results screen looked all blurry, and they just appeared to me, as if they shone out, the expressions "carcinoma is a type of cancer that starts in cells..." and "like other types of cancer, carcinomas are cells that develop without control...".

Honestly, I find it difficult to express with words a moment like that, which I don't want for anyone. I believe that no person does not feel a profound impact on the revelation that she has cancer. Trying to revisit that instant, I can't describe the feeling. It is one of the moments in life that I will never forget. I surely will not.

That Monday, September 2, 2019, will never be forgotten by me, until the end of life. I don't know if it's my imagination or if it's real, but it seems that one of the thoughts that crossed my mind was one of relief, because at least this kind of ritual would come to an end, would end. What comforted me was the possibility of having a diagnosis at the beginning of the development of the disease and that the probability of cure, in this case, would be very high. On the other hand, this issue of a high likelihood of healing is very relative for those who have the disease, I will comment on that in the next chapter.

I remember well that I thought about how I would tell my wife and son. Then I thought of my father, tell him or not? He's already been through this, should I tell him? It's strange how such an impacting moment can leave feelings so blurry in the memory and felt so deeply in the guts.

Well, the ritual had to continue.

The next step was to return to the doctor and define

the treatment, which from what I had already informed myself, would probably be a surgery of total removal of the prostate.

In the return visit, there was another remarkable moment. It was only two days between the science for the report and the consultation. The doctor had already received the result directly from the laboratory, so he asked me if I had read it. Yes, I already knew the result, I told him.

Even so, he followed the protocol, explaining the result, and in the end, speaking the expression "...is cancer". Even if I already knew, it was impressive to hear that.

A score called Gleason depicts the results report of a prostate biopsy.

It is quite complicated for a layman like me to explain, but to summarize, it is a score between 2 and 10, and a score of up to 6 can be considered low grade. Seven is deemed to be intermediate and, between 8 and 10, high degree, or high-aggression cancer.

According to the biopsy, I had a Gleason 7 (3+4).

The 7 of my examinations resulted from 3 + 4 (which is a different result than the 7 resulting from 4 + 3). The doctor explained that it was a medium intensity cancer, and according to the other parameters stated by the report, theoretically would be contained, restricted to the prostate, and probably would not have affected other external tissues.

The conclusion is that, among the worst results, this was the least bad. I mean, if it was Gleason 6 or less, maybe it wasn't even necessary to treat, it could just be followed up (when he said this, I thought to myself, *"I'm glad it's not six because the affliction would persist for longer"*).

But!

A comprehensive explanation followed it. Even with the complete removal of the prostate and seminal vesicles, being the nodules restricted and contained (there were three tumors in fact), there was a probability that some cells may have "escaped" into the bloodstream and contaminated some other tissue. Contamination would mean leaving some cancer residue even after the complete removal. In this case, the sequence of treatment should be radiotherapy.

That's when I thought to myself: *"I don't believe it, does that mean that not even taking everything out of the nightmare will end?"*. I didn't count on this one, because I was already preparing myself to face the surgery (even with the fear of possible sequelae) and soon after be free. I was downcast and a lot.

For clarification, the doctor presented the treatment options, one of them being radiotherapy instead of removal surgery. It is a less radical process than the total removal of the prostate. Still, it is more prolonged, uncertain, subject to the same risks, and also without guaranteed results.

The recommendation that I got, a standard for patients at my age, was for surgery, although the final decision on treatment was mine.

I opted for surgery, and fortunately for the circumstances, I was able to choose robotic technology, which is less invasive, reducing recovery time and reducing the risk of sequelae.

And the risks, what are they?

Risks were made very clear in this consultation, clarified in a very formally, but empathetic way. There are two significant risks, urinary incontinence (and the need to use diapers) and sexual impotence, also called erectile dysfunction. The first is due to the urethra being "reconnected" to the bladder next to the sphincter. The second risk may result from the possibility of affecting a nerve responsible for erection. Let's agree that for men, none of these perspectives is reassuring.

Anyway, the ritual wasn't over yet. Before the surgery, four preoperative exams are necessary, two CT scans (from abdomen and thorax), bone scintigraphy, and blood exams, besides a consultation to obtain a cardiologist's certificate. The CT scans try to identify if any organ presents any alteration, and bone scintigraphy seeks to evaluate if there is any suspicion of bone cancer.

With the confirmation of cancer, a heavy burden, there were two new waits for reports that tested to the limit my mental resistance.

Imagine, reader, thinking about the possibility of having a metastasis to the bones or the lung. It's very frightening. Fortunately, in my case, these new tests were negative. At one point, I thought it was a relief to have only prostate cancer. In a way, it was.

* * *

From the moment I became aware of the confirmation of cancer, I cannot describe the feeling. I went into a kind of awake hibernation, even though I tried to continue with an ordinary life, going to work, going to the gym, doing weight training and running. It seems that sometimes I saw the world go by in slow motion, sometimes it gave a strange sensation of not being able to connect with the present. It's very complicated to describe. Still, there is a moment when it seems that one is taken by thought in such a way that no other sense works appropriately. Thinking about the surgery, the possible sequelae, what could go wrong. And if all goes well, when would life return to normal?

It's a huge burden. At this time, the ghost has become a demon.

WAYS TO FACE CANCER

I don't think there's any easy way to face a cancer diagnosis. It is impossible, therefore, that this subject does not become almost omnipresent in thoughts when the person is faced with the real possibility of diagnosing cancer. Of course, with the confirmed diagnosis too.

> *Things are always going through our minds, some of them rational, others unreasonable, on the brink of the absurd. Actually, I don't believe that anyone can live an ordinary life knowing they have cancer.*

I tried to rationalize that there is always some probability that cells get out of control and start to reproduce at random. Never mind that I thought that this can happen to any human being. Still, it was inevitable that I would ask myself: "why me?"

In my case, prostate cancer, the fact that my father had the disease automatically turned me into an attention patient. As soon as my PSA level was detected as abnormal for my age (just over 40 years old), I started a more intensive follow-up. Even though there is no standard for what can be considered high, in general, the expected level for young men is below 1. As at the time my result was above 1, according to science and the law of probabilities, I knew I should prepare for this possibility.

I always thought I was preparing myself. On second thought, I even think I've always been at least considering a possible fatality. On the day that my PSA level increased a little more sharply, I started an investigation following the traditional steps of the ritual - ultrasound, MRI, and biopsy. I realized then that no preparation had been enough. There was always a kind of arms fall between me knowing that it could happen and forgetting not to suffer in advance.

Once a negative diagnosis was confirmed, it was better not to think about it until next year - or next semester. I tried to forget it, but sometimes I couldn't. It's funny, but I forgot without forgetting. From time to time, there was news that an acquaintance had been diagnosed with cancer, and that was it, the ghosts would come back. After a short time, they would go.

I don't know how to define it, but this wasn't a real burden, life went on regularly. It was more like a small stone in the shoe, so tiny that every now and then, it disappears without being removed.

* * *

A contradictory feeling that came to my mind when it was confirmed that I had cancer was related to a supposed high probability of cure. It is often heard that prostate cancer, when discovered in the beginning, has a high likelihood of healing, something like 95%. For people who see from the outside, this seems a very reassuring statistic, there appears to be no reason to worry, after all, only 5% of the cases cannot be cured. When I heard about my father's cancer, that's exactly how I thought. Having the disease and fearing to become a statistical occurrence among the 5%, I can guarantee that the tranquility is not so great.

I can give an example with an analogy, through a simple question for you, dear reader: if the statistics showed that 5% of flights suffered air accidents, would you fly? Why not? It's a 95% chance of nothing happening...

* * *

Out of rationality, some ridiculously absurd thoughts appeared:

Was cancer some karma?

Payment for some guilt?

A punishment?

I do not intend to divert to this esoteric side, because it is not my intention to approach the question of faith or religion. Not because I underestimate or not believe, but to keep the focus on feelings, thoughts, and the timeline that unfolded from the investigation to the treatment.

To put it on record, anyway, I don't think it's a punishment or that I've deserved to go through it.

Nobody deserves

EXPECTATION IS DIFFERENT FROM REALITY

I f we leave the disease aside for a moment, it is consistent with admitting that often, what is expected of something is different from reality.

This is true for practically everything in life, bad things, and also for the right things. Who hasn't waited too long for something that then, when it happened, wasn't what you imagined? There are plenty of examples, it could have been a school excursion, a party, a trip, a courtship, etc. In short, surely everyone must remember something that, in reality, turned out to be quite different from what was expected.

The fact is, in a horrible case, such as cancer, the same happens. I imagined that I was preparing for the inevitable. Even I were rationalizing and projecting how I would feel, it didn't come close to how the real feeling was when the cancer was confirmed. Not even close.

> *I confess that I felt the blow; it took me several days even to be able to say the phrase "I have cancer," because, for a while, this did not seem real. The projection about pain does not mean feeling it, reality hurts much more.*

Less harm than the opposite is also true; that is, the memory about pain does not reproduce the intensity in which it was felt.

FEAR AND DENIAL

I believe that being human means, among other things, being afraid. It is impossible that someone has never had it or does not have it.

According to one of the generic definitions, fear is "an emotional state provoked by the consciousness that one has in the face of danger; that which provokes that consciousness." As I wrote earlier, I believe in a kind of collective fear of cancer. Well, why are people afraid of cancer? For two reasons, fear of suffering and fear of dying. It is inevitable to associate the disease with both.

Among all human feelings, fear is perhaps one of the most tormenting. It can become omnipotent, it really paralyzes a person, no matter how much one tries to rationalize to fight it. There is no magic formula for overcoming fear. Still, one way that can prove useful for the unconscious is to deny, to deny that there are a threat and danger.

This is what crossed my mind countless times as I feared to have cancer, and then when I confirmed that I had it.

More than once, I found myself thinking that maybe the material of my exams had been changed. That the results report had my name by mistake. That the tissue samples of my biopsy had been changed. I really expected that there was some mistake in some procedures and that I had no cancer.

The mind, threatened by fear, tries anyway to get rid of the threat. Countless times, I found myself denying the situation.

IT IS COOL NOT TO BE AFRAID

I have heard that the human being is the only species that is aware of the inevitability of death. Yet, we all know or hear about people who are not afraid to die.

Some people are not afraid of height, while others are. Some are not afraid of planes, while others cannot even get into one. I do not know if I can say that I admire those who are not afraid because the particularities of individual experiences are not comparable. I don't think it's any big deal that I'm not scared to fly, nor do I think it's anything less than that someone has that phobia. Thoughts and feelings have no scale and are not comparable.

* * *

We live in the age of appearances, amplified by social networks. Publicly most people seem to lead a perfect life. This is a proven thesis of psychological and sociological studies, taking a certain amount of anguish to some people who are constantly comparing themselves to those who have a "beautiful life."

We all have different perceptions of reality, right? When it comes to feelings and their intensity, we don't even talk, because they are subjective and determined by the sum of individual attributes of each one. The way we react to the facts of life is part of the personality and experiences of being of each one.

It is probable, therefore, that many men have had the experience of discovering prostate cancer without having felt even a fraction of what I felt. To them, my feelings and fears certainly sound exaggerated, perhaps they think I am being dramatic. Maybe they're right.

I don't think about comparing and dare not feel from the perspective of right or wrong. My feelings were of fear, anguish, and impatience, even if I did not prefer to feel that way. I don't think there are any wrong feelings.

Sometimes I found myself thinking about whether or not I was playing the victim or exaggerating in the drama. Incredible as it may seem, it sometimes even generated guilt.

Indeed, this attitude was not verbally shared with other people. It was a matter of thought - further on, I will address this question of how to relate to family and other people.

OPPRESSIVE RECURRENT THINKING

Being aware that one has cancer is not something that can be filed in a drawer in the warehouse of the unconscious to gather dust. No matter what one tries to do to be distracted, busy with life, filling time with work or leisure activities: thinking about cancer insists on returning to the surface frequently.

* * *

Whether in the middle of a meeting or focused on some intellectual venture, out of nowhere came to mind a luminous and audible 'shit, I have cancer' warning.

Watching a movie, running, drinking a glass of good wine, listening to music, or reading a book, in some moments of distraction, it seemed that life was beautiful. Suddenly, out of nowhere, the alert popped up. When it appeared, it was like a cold water bath, a nuisance that reminded me again that life did not follow its usual course.

The thought is powerful. If there is one thing I couldn't do was not think about cancer. There are classic examples of this, it would be the same as what I now say to you, reader, not to think about a horse. I bet you thought of a horse!

The difference is that the memory of cancer is not something accessory in anyone's life, it is a thought that is recurrent, it becomes oppressive. It ends up sucking in a lot of energy.

It's exhausting.

WHAT IS HOPE?

I wrote about fear, denial, dysfunctional, and oppressive thoughts. It is the reality that I experienced in a difficult period of reflection that led me to another conclusion:

Just as the human being is the only one with an awareness of death, I believe he is the only one who can (or needs) to wait for things to improve.

Waiting for things to improve led me to think about what it means to hope, or to believe.

It seems to me that all can be defined by two words, hope, and faith, although both seem to be the same thing. I'm not sure if they are different. Still, if they are, maybe it's because the latter bears spiritual, esoteric, or religion-related beliefs. Hope is similar, or the same thing, except that it is not only on the religious side. However, it is still mysterious.

I have seen cases of people in situations of terminal illness who did not lose hope. Even in a dire state, they hoped only to be able to spend their next Christmas with their families. What faith! The human being's adaptation to adversities is impressive.

Perhaps the highest awareness I have acquired as a result of the experience I have lived is that it is impossible to live without hope, or without faith, as you wish.

HOW TO DEAL WITH THE FAMILY

Obviously, this is not a question for which there is a ready answer or a formula. It depends on the condition of each individual concerning their family structure and the group of people closest to them.

I have always shared with my wife and son information about the stages of the ritual, informing about what would be evaluated in each exam, the results that would be expected (or not), and the confirmed diagnoses. I can't say precisely how they felt. Still, the reactions have always been to verbalize support in the best way that people can, saying that I shouldn't worry and that everything would work out.

In "good" diagnostic situations, there was obviously a general relief, and life took its course. Soon after the last diagnosis of a PSA with very significant variation, the last one that culminated in the confirmation of cancer, we made an enjoyable trip on a family vacation, totally ignoring the prospects of the scenario that might lie ahead.

On the day I had the MRI scan result that indicated a very high suspicion of cancer (that of PIRADS-4), I remember that the impact on them was tremendous. It was not something explicit or verbalized, but I could tell by the non-verbal language.

With this, as incredible as it may seem, a new feeling emerged in me, which was absurd, but real: guilt.

It took me a while to realize, but I analyzed it and realized that deep down, I felt bad for making them go through it. As irrational and unfair as it sounds, that's what I felt, I had to work on it when seeking professional help (I'll talk more ahead about the importance that psychic help support brought me).

I was transparent with them, I exposed the situation. Obviously, the shock happened, I realized clearly. With the confirmation of the diagnosis of cancer, I understood that I developed some conflicts:

From then on, how should I act?

Don't touch on the subject and pretend that nothing was happening?

Always try to represent that I was well, even in my worst moments?

Or keep touching on the subject repeatedly, fearing of not letting them forget the issue?

There is no right recipe, I used to say some things when I felt the need to talk, and my wife expressed a concern in a very appropriate way, neither too much nor too little, her attitude showing affection and kind support.

My son, a young adult, is more closed, avoid touching the subject directly with me, asked little, more because it is a personal characteristic of him, of course.

My wife told me that they talked a lot about it and that he was obviously distraught. I believe that I did my part because I always tried to keep them informed and aware of the whole process.

I also had doubts about telling my father or not, once he had already gone through this situation and is a certain advanced age. I thought about sparing him the bad news, but at the same time, I imagined that I wanted my son to share his difficulties with me so that I could support him.

It took me a while to decide, I exchanged ideas with my sister, and we concluded together that he should know. Since I don't live in the same city as my father, the task was left to her, who volunteered to tell in person (they live nearby each other). Surprisingly, according to her, he reacted very well, called me soon after she heard, and supported me to a very adequate extent. My conclusion is that I ended up doing him right by allowing him to help me.

For those who live in a cancer situation, personal relationships are complicated to balance. There are times when you can forget about the disease, but when someone comes to ask how you are, obviously, it is a memory that comes back just at a moment that you had forgotten. On the other hand, when the interest is genuine, the right is full and justifiable.

On the other hand, if I felt like talking about it, it could be provoking a negative memory in people when they had forgotten the subject.

What, then, is the best way to deal with the family?

There is no better way, or if there is, I haven't found out. I indeed found a way, privately, to deal with the situation without talking to people all the time. The move was to write. During the journey, I wrote a lot of notes and records of feelings that resulted in this book. As I have already commented, it was an excellent tool for personal catharsis, as if I were talking to myself so as not to disturb others.

HOW TO BEHAVE IN PUBLIC

The considerations in the previous chapter were about my family. Still, another doubt I had was how I would feel better to deal with the situation than other people in my life, including those at work.

Because of my personality and personal choice, which was well resolved, I consider myself to be reserved and, even to some extent, introverted. Introversion is different from shyness, I am not shy, I just choose to be, as is popularly said, "more reserved" and not expose intimacies. It does not mean that I judge or find inappropriate those who act differently. Still, I do not usually share in social networks, for example, personal things.

Due to my way of being, I felt a significant doubt about telling or not others about my cancer.

My choice was not to talk about the disease with everyone with whom I had some contact, much less share it on social networks.

I decided to restrict the "disclosure" to a few people. To those with a direct relationship at work. To those who would be impacted by my absence due to the treatment. To some others with whom some appointments would eventually have to be postponed. All of this was due to the marathon of exams and preparations for the surgery and the surgery itself.

On the other hand, I didn't ask anyone to keep it a secret; after all, it wasn't something I needed to hide.

As I have previously written, the thought about the disease is somewhat omnipresent in all directions, which included not only me about the others but also the others about me.

I remember when I talked to people, deep down, I kept trying to guess whether they knew about my illness or not. I believe that those who knew were also a little doubtful about how to behave toward me, whether they should bring it up or not. Maybe they even felt some kind of empathy mixed with a feeling of relief, like "what a f***, I didn't want to be in his shoes...".

LOOKING FOR PROFESSIONAL HELP

In this last cycle of the journey, the one that culminated in the confirmation of the diagnosis of cancer, I made a decision that helped me a lot. I sought help from a mental health professional, a psychiatrist.

It seems to me that this is another unspoken taboo in our society: a man does not need a psychologist, or especially a psychiatrist. That is something for a mentally ill or a nut.

I had psychotherapy for a long time with a psychiatrist; it helped a lot in my self-knowledge and the solution of some neuroses, which improved a lot my quality of life.

In this specific case of cancer, however, I did not seek psychotherapy, but rather a prompt, behavioral, and mainly oriented support to deal with the anxiety arising from the situation. The professional I consulted is a psychiatrist specialized in anxiety and *Cognitive Behavioral Therapy* (CBT).

Probably due to the emotional pressure to which I was submitted, added to the other vicissitudes of modern life, my diagnosis was of a principle of depression. I don't know for sure, but maybe some people feel embarrassed to say that they have depression.

I have always been resistant to taking medication, and it was no different in this case. I ended up convinced by the psychiatrist that, given the circumstances, it would be better for me to take an antidepressant drug. I was reluctant but accepted. Although I was also told to use anxiolytics moderately, I never used them, except once before the last MRI. I use to say that my best anxiolytic is jogging.

In a few sessions and with the support of appropriate medications, I felt that my emotional state improved a lot. I am convinced that I supported the whole process with much more stability of emotions and mental resilience.

Cognitive Behavioral Therapy has helped a lot with techniques to shift from catastrophic dysfunctional thinking to focus on possible positive scenarios and to exercise preparation for eventual unwanted situations. Exercises supported by methods helped to achieve this. Together with the support of the medication, I felt better.

In practice, what has happened is that the intensity of negative and catastrophic thoughts has dramatically decreased, along with anxiety. Of course, after everything that is terrible passes, it seems that it was not so unpleasant. Still, it is essential to point out that the possible functional scenarios that I was exercising ended up happening. If I had had the ability, I would have liked to have been less worried, and I would have achieved the same result.

I wrote at the beginning, and it is essential to remember that my goal is not to offer self-help tips. Still, if I had to highlight some suggestions for those who will go through this situation, it would undoubtedly be: seek professional help for mental stability. It will decrease your anxiety, your anguish, your suffering.

RESIGNATION AND A NEW MARATHON: SURGERY

I came this far going through what I called the diagnostic ritual, facing fatality, denying it, feeling anxiety, fear, and hope. Then at some point in my journey, I was sure that I had cancer. Now, it was the time to perform the treatment, for which I opted for radical prostatectomy. It is a surgery which means to remove the prostate, the seminal vesicles, and section the canal that takes the spermatozoa to the penis. Surgery and recovery, for me, represented a real marathon, after the diagnostic journey.

Before the surgery itself, the marathon started. Several pre-surgical exams are necessary, comprising 2 CT scans (of the abdomen and chest), bone scintigraphy, blood and urine exams, and also a consultation with a cardiologist to obtain a certificate.

The CT scans seek to identify if any organ presents alterations that suggest a tumor, while bone scintigraphy aims to evaluate if there is any suspicion of bone cancer. It is worth remembering something I described in the chapter about the importance of diagnosis, that this would be the manifestation of metastasis.

With a confirmed diagnosis of cancer and the exponentially higher emotional pressure, I faced two new waits for reports that tested my mental resistance to the limit. Imagine thinking about the possibility of not only having prostate cancer but having a metastasis to the bones or the lung!

It's not something for amateurs in the area of mental endurance and emotional control.

Fortunately, in my case, these new tests did not result in unwanted diagnoses. At one point, relieved, I came to think that I was lucky to have only one prostate cancer. And on second thought, it was.

❊ ❊ ❊

As fortunately, I always had good health. For me, the routine of a hospital was unknown, let alone that of surgery. With the date confirmed, there was nothing left to do but resign me and focus on the pre-surgical exams that were necessary. And then try to forget everything until the last day arrived.

I managed to schedule the surgery for about three weeks after the diagnosis was confirmed. Scheduling surgery requires an alignment of the doctor's schedule, his team, and the hospital operating room. Three weeks was a very tight time, given the need to schedule and perform the pre-surgical exams (which, moreover, required submission for approval of my health plan). I tried to do it this way, as soon as possible, because I wanted to end everything immediately. I spent a long time planning (scheduling) and performing all the exams in about two weeks.

Fortunately, I got all the reports and the cardiologist's certificate in this short period. I confess that I spent a lot of time in the planning and execution of this endeavor so that everything would fit together.

As the day of the surgery approached, I felt strangely calm, part by the result of the depression treatment and part by the imminence that soon everything would end. I decided to do my best not to let myself down. As preparation support, I intensified the joggings, and I kept going to the gym, confident that the physical well-being would help in the recovery.

I could write a lot about the wonders that running provides, among them, as in my case, anxiety control (as I usually repeat, it is my natural Rivotril). As

I ran a lot in the period before the surgery, I was very well prepared physically, which later proved to be very useful for recovery.

* * *

As I have already mentioned, I opted for surgery, which is called radical prostatectomy and can be performed by the surgeon in three different ways. The "traditional" way. By video laparoscopy. In some cases, where the technology is available, with the support of robotic technology, performed by the *Da Vinci robot*, one of the most advanced surgical resources in the world.

> *Robotics increases surgical precision, is less invasive, and, therefore, reduces blood loss and the likelihood of sequelae, in addition to reducing recovery time (with consequent shorter hospitalization time).*

Some may be wondering why then everyone would not always opt for this more advanced possibility if it is the best choice in all aspects. Everyone should do it, but there are some obstacles. In the first place, it is a new technology, costly and still restricted to large centers. As a consequence, due to the high investment cost, it is an expensive procedure. Some health insurance plans do not provide coverage. I have a good one, but it did not provide coverage for the choice to use the robot.

Given my history and my condition of risk, I had taken out insurance coverage for serious illnesses - cancer among them. This decision gave me peace of mind in dealing with this financial issue.

One recommendation I dare give is that readers be informed about the feasibility of taking out cancer treatment insurance. Of course, this depends on one's financial condition, but it doesn't cost to evaluate the possibility.

Whichever method of surgery I would choose, one fact worried me too much. For recovery, it would be necessary to have a catheter entering the penile canal, directly connected to the bladder. It would be for seven days, or maybe more.

* * *

The surgery

On the day of the operation, I arrived earlier at the hospital. No special preparation was necessary, except for an 8-hour fast due to general anesthesia.

After check-in, I waited for a little. I was soon called to the operating room, when I changed my clothes for the apron and waited for an interview with the anesthesiologist, for protocol questions, general guidelines, and clarification of doubts that I had. At this moment, a relative was allowed to enter, and I had the company of my wife.

Then, there was a new wait of about one hour (sincerely I was strangely calm), until they called me again. I said goodbye to my wife and my son, who was outside the door of the surgery block.

I entered the operating room, walking. There was the doctor and his staff, including the anesthesiologist. The atmosphere was very relaxed, and I met the robot, which reminded me of a mechanical science fiction film spider with its metal claws. I lay on the table still quietly, and shortly after, they started the intravenous anesthesia. When they put the oxygen mask over my nose and mouth, I completely fell asleep.

❊ ❊ ❊

As the light came on, I opened my eyes in the recovery room, the one with the curtains separating the beds. A nurse was there asking my name, my date of birth, and if I was okay. I answered and soon went out again.

As I woke up later, with no idea how much time had passed, I saw my wife and son by the bedside. I even managed to say a few words, but I remember it was challenging. Only then did I realize that I had a kind of electric massager involving both legs, which made continuous massage movements. With difficulty, I asked the nurse what it was when she told me it was a mechanism to avoid embolism. With the internal bleeding caused by the surgery, there was a risk of clotting some blood vessels.

Almost instantly, even though I felt that lethargy, I remembered the catheter. I had already been informed by the doctor that I would have a tube directly in the bladder, with the hose entering through the penis for at least seven days.

OMG, the catheter!

I lifted the apron to check, looked, and there it was, the confirmation of my concern, my inseparable company, for the next few days. I had another strange thought at that moment. I don't know where it came from, and I wondered if maybe that was a dream and that I would wake up in my bed at home. Unfortunately, it was not.

At that moment, I felt two things: sleepiness and nausea. They gave me water to drink and something to eat, and I couldn't, the nausea was extreme. I believe it was about 4 hours before they took me to my room, after waking up with an intense sweat and a horrible sensation of not-know-what. Later my son told me that I was as white as the bedsheets.

* * *

I remember the feeling of the bed pushed through the corridors and elevators, a typical image of films in which a lying patient only sees the ceiling and the lights that pass over his eyes. Even with the slow movement of the bed, the nausea was extreme.

Pain?

I was under some residual effect of the anesthesia and with three types of painkillers given every three hours, one of them injected into the vein. Even so, I felt severe pain in my throat. They told me that it was a result of the "intubation" of the general anesthesia. Besides the pain in the throat, I still felt nausea and tiredness.

They took me to my room at about 1 a.m. I chose to be alone, and I insisted that no one in the family stay in the hospital.

Another severe pain began to appear when I cough. Due to the throat injury, a permanent irritation caused an intermittent cough, extreme by the way. In those moments, the pain became very intense, due to the impacting movement that the cough causes in the abdomen.

The next day, early in the morning, I was helped by nurses to get out of bed and take some steps around the room. They told me that this was important to help with my recovery. For safety reasons, because it was the first time I got up, it had to be in their presence.

In the afternoon, I got out of bed again, by myself, and I was able to walk a little longer. About 24 hours after the surgery, I even took a few steps down the corridor of the hospital (taking with me, of course, with the urine bag).

There is one detail that I must record, a significant discomfort that I felt as a result of robotic surgery. Some amount of carbon dioxide is injected into the abdomen, to make the procedure more manageable, which makes it very "swollen." Swelling causes an uncomfortable sensation, because it restricts the lung space, giving the impression that one cannot breathe properly. It looks like as if it were not possible to fill the entire lung with air.

On the second day after the surgery, I continued to walk around, spending most of the time out of bed. As I was feeling better, I began to feel the boredom of hospitalization.

On the third day, I asked not to take more oral painkillers, because I felt stomach irritation with the medicines. As a result, I began to feel an inevitable constant pain in my abdomen, which was bearable for me. The pain was preferable to aggression to my stomach - the situation only got worse even when I coughed. It was a pain similar to the muscular pain I felt when I exaggerated in abdominal exercises - although much more intense.

This day I had help from a physiotherapist who guided me with breathing exercises (due to the compression of the lung caused by the gas in the abdomen). She also helped me with the basic movements of muscular activation and stretching. According to her, my recovery was being excellent, which leads me to believe that focusing on physical preparation before surgery was a wise decision.

A suggestion that I can give without fear of making a mistake is that physical preparation is crucial when someone goes through a surgical procedure.

At that point, I was feeling ready to go home.

At night, during the doctor's visit, it was agreed that if no unexpected event arose, the next day I would be discharged from hospital.

And so it was, the third day after the surgery, I was ready to go home.

As expected, the decision for robotic surgery proved to be the best choice. I had a relatively fast recovery, which is is a result of the greater precision and smaller invasion of the procedure. There were four small incisions of about 1.5 inches and one of about 3 inches, at most - all in the abdomen.

I have to confess, three days in a hospital were already driving me crazy! In addition to confinement, the routine of nurses' interventions every three hours, even during the night, makes sleep difficult. Not to mention that the catheter already showed the one that was coming, I began to notice the size of the inconvenience that the new companion would bring me for a whole week.

The truth is: it is very uncomfortable.

On discharge day, the hospital's support staff took me in a wheelchair to the parking lot ("house rules"). I felt strange, just four days before I was running in the park with a performance from someone well prepared physically. Still, now I felt exhausted and being pushed into the chair with a urine bag hanging from it.

HOME, SWEET HOME. AND THE DESIRED DIVORCE

ome at last!

I left the hospital around noon. That same afternoon, and still at night, the hospital had not left me, I smelled and heard the noises of the hospital routine. When I tried to sleep, I had the feeling that a nurse would enter my bedroom every three hours. To make matters worse, I felt intense pain when I coughed.

The next day the situation improved, I was finally able to feel at home. My inseparable companion, the catheter, continued with me.

I was adapting fast to coexistence, and I began to architect ways to accommodate her next to me to sit down, lie down on the couch, take a bath, and also in the physiological necessities.

It is incredible how the human being adapts well to the difficulties. In a short time, I had the support points to hang it wherever I was in my routine of domestic hospitalization. It was as if I had an anchor launched wherever I went.

It was challenging to sleep, especially as I was afraid to pull the catheter out involuntarily. I ended up finding a curious way to feel safe, with a tape of that kind of paper for paint insulation: I attached the catheter hose to my thigh with the tape, which gave me more confidence so I wouldn't have any sudden pulling.

The bath wasn't comfortable either, because I had to hold the hose with one hand and wash with the other. I needed help from my wife to get it.

On the third day at home (the fifth day after the surgery,) I went for a walk on the treadmill, at a slow pace, is true, for about 15 minutes. Guess what? With my integral partner in my hand, of course. At that time, our relationship was beginning to deteriorate, and it was starting to turn into hatred.

It was only two days before the catheter go. On the eve before the removal, influenced psychologically by the imminent prospect of freedom, that thing began to be an enormous nuisance. I tried not to think about it, but it was inevitable:

There are 26 hours left.

Tomorrow, at this time, I will be retiring.

In 14 hours I'll be free.

Finally, the day came! I didn't sleep much the night before, and I woke up early. I couldn't stay in bed, after all, *there were only 7 hours left!*

AN UNFORGETTABLE DAY

This day will be one of the most unforgettable of all my life, for everything he represented. Not only because of the divorce with the catheter. I had an enormous expectation about what the next days would be like regarding the rest of my life.

I have already written about the risks of surgery, one of which is urinary incontinence. For medical advice, I was advised to take a male absorbent to the appointment for the removal of the catheter(I confess, I didn't even know this existed!). I don't believe that any adult is indifferent to the possibility of having to wear diapers.

Last but not least, it was the day of knowing the result of the pathological analysis of all the material extracted. It is essential to clarify that everything removed in the surgery, including the prostate itself and some adjacent tissues, is sent to a laboratory for pathological analysis. That analysis will confirm the type of tumor cells and, more importantly, the coverage of these cells and the containment or not of cancer. The result of this examination may indicate the likelihood that cancer is completely removed or that some carcinogenic tissue has remained in the body.

If any tissue outside the prostate had these cells, the cure would not be complete, and a radiotherapy treatment should then be required.

In short, this was a day when I would have an immense relief and at the same time, expecting a very, very important result.

Could it be more unforgettable?

Finally, the consultation arrived; the removal of the catheter occurs in the doctor's office. The procedure is straightforward; all the doctor does is "pull the hose." It's very uncomfortable, but it doesn't hurt. After all, it's an absurdly expected moment. The first thing I did, free of my partner, was to get out of the office bed and walk around the room.

What a good feeling!

At that moment, in the office, there was no "leakage"

of urine. The doctor guided me on how to use the absorbent, and I left the office "protected" by one. According to him, it would be reasonable for me to need this protection in the next few days until I regained control. I would need to be careful, especially when coughing, standing up, and performing some other sudden movements.

In some situations, it may be necessary to deal with incontinence for weeks or even months - each case is a case, he explained to me.

When I asked about the pathological result, he told me that he had not yet received it, would call me as soon as he had it. I asked him which laboratory would analyze the material. It was the same one that examined the content of the last biopsy.

* * *

I got home, and, of course, my thinking was about urination. I felt nothing different about being wet, and I often checked the absorbent, which was dry.

A couple of hours later, full of expectation, I had my first experience of urinating directly in the toilet, standing up. With a gratifying feeling, everything went well. What do I mean by everything going well?

I pissed like I always did in life!

I felt a bit of burning. Still, according to the doctor, this could be expected since the catheter could cause contamination with urinary infection (I had an antibiotic prescription, which is a standard procedure).

In the upcoming events of a visit to the bathroom, although the burning remained, everything continued to go well. The most incredible thing is that the next morning, the absorbent was still dry, so I decided not to use it anymore.

In other words: I left a prostatectomy surgery without even a day of loss of urinary control. Not to mention that I was 100% the same as before the surgery, I realized that when doing the "number 2" need simultaneously get out a little "number 1", which is not the standard physiology.

✳ ✳ ✳

I can't help but comment on the wonder of sleeping free from the catheter, not to mention the bath.

How beautiful those moments were.

No matter how cliché this sounds, how simple things have value when you lose so little of normality in life.

AN UNFORGETTABLE EVENING

It was very uncomfortable for me to share personal issues, such as those I have reported so far. I must confess, therefore, that it took me a long time to convince myself to include this chapter in the book. I ended up giving in to the conclusion that without it, the story would not be complete, or rather, there would be an open gap without the proper clarification, with outstanding doubts.

Let's get to the point. The third night I slept at home, I had a surprise, which was not, fortunately, waking up urinated.

When I woke up from a deep sleep, very probably from the REM stage, I realized that I had a partial erection. All of us, men, know that this is normal.

Still, considering the situation I was in, uncertain about the result of the surgery about this aspect, it was even comical.

I was pleased!

At the same time, I ended up with considerable doubt. Could an involuntary sleep erection have anything to do with the fact that all erectile functions were intact? I admit that I was ignorant about the subject (it was more of a learning experience that I ended up absorbing when I experienced the situations).

A very strange Whatsapp message

The next day I woke up early, eager to clear up my doubts. It was then that I sent a WhatsApp message to my doctor, explaining the situation and asking if this event was a good sign. I confess that I found it a bit strange to send a message to another man talking about an erection. Even today, I find it funny, by the way.

What about his answer?

"That was a great sign."

Well, that's as much as I can share intimacy in this area.

In a very general way, I can say that right after that I was able to test my reactions to certain "physiological stimuli." I confirmed that the result couldn't be better.

THE FINAL SPRINT

Everything was going too well. The marathon was in the final sprint, only the result of the pathology exam was missing. I wouldn't be comfortable waiting for a phone call to find out the result.

I called the laboratory directly as I had done at the time of the biopsy and asked them to send me the report by e-mail when it was ready. This way I wouldn't depend on the doctor's call, as he is swamped and does many surgeries. I didn't want to run the risk of being notified a time after the report was available).

At the call, the laboratory attendant informed me that the report was ready. Still, there was no signature from the doctor in charge, which would only happen the next day. I already had at that time an individual experience with this type of procedure, and I didn't even try to ask her to send me the report without a signature. I knew what the answer would be - this is probably not allowed for legal reasons. Incredible, my destiny was in front of her, on the other side of the line, but I couldn't know the result.

Another day of waiting.

> For those who have expected so many reports that would determine so much, what was to wait another day?

What would it be like to spend another night not knowing about another vital result?

At last, the next day arrived.

I was in the final sprint of a marathon, seeing the finish line just ahead.

> Try to imagine, dear reader, the sensation: either I would be free from the nightmare, in paradise, or I would have to face another frustration, then join forces and continue fighting against cancer, with the uncertainties and risks of another type of treatment. In other words, I would remain in hell.

All determined by an e-mail!

On this day, nothing made me stop checking the e-mails, sometimes on the computer, sometimes on the cell phone.

I updated inbox all the time, refresh, refresh, refresh, refresh. What I wanted to see didn't show up.

Then the e-mail showed up!

When I accessed the report, I read everything I wanted:

- The Gleason 7 (3+4) detected in the biopsy was confirmed, meaning that the tumor was no worse than it looked.

- The tumor occupied approximately 15% of the prostate volume.

- The tumor was inside the prostate, and all surrounding tissues were free of neoplasia.

At this moment, I think I had an outbreak of adrenaline overload. I started to walk restlessly through my home, I even thought about opening the window and screaming, I was extremely agitated, not knowing what to do. It was one of the most memorable moments of my entire life.

It was the morning of October 2, 2019, and
the journey ended 72 days after it began.

72 DAYS FROM HELL TO HEAVEN

Since the result of the last much more altered PSA exam until I crossed the finish line, it has been 72 days.

Eight days passed between surgery and recovery, including hospital stay, living with a catheter, and the expectation of a pathological result related to the healing or not of cancer.

I had never had the opportunity to stop to think so much about what a few days can represent in people's lives. I have been living at a pace that swallows months as if they were weeks, with a perception that the years are passing very fast; it seems that it was just the turn of the year, and it is almost Christmas again! In the next few years, I have the impression that it will look even faster.

I believe this is not just my feeling.

With time passing at this speed, what are eight days, what are 72 days?

On a tourist trip and holidays, eight days fly.

Professionally, I usually get involved in projects that have their stages planned in weeks or months, with deadlines (almost always) tight, a situation in which the days and weeks fly. In these circumstances, 72 days pass very fast.

It is impressive, however, how the relativity of time has been noticed, for example, in the mere seven days in which I lived with the catheter for at least three reasons.

The first reason is because of the physical limitation and mechanical discomfort of the situation. Everything, absolutely everything, is limited with a hose on the penis connected to a bag. Moving around, sleeping, bathing, everything that is done mechanically in regular times, becomes more complicated. The sensation is also bizarre because the bag receives the drip of urine permanently, and the brain, used to be activated to trigger the need to urinate, becomes confused. When performing the physiological need of "number 2", it is even stranger, because there is no sphincter control for urine and everything is very confusing.

Secondly, but no less impactful, due to the impatience for the removal of the catheter to then acknowledge how things would look. It is impossible not to think about the perspective (or hope) of regaining control over the bladder if this would happen to the satisfaction. It was a period in which I was emotionally weakened, and with it, the dysfunctional thoughts gain strength.

The third reason, equally considerable, is the waiting for the definitive pathological report on the analysis of all the material removed - the prostate itself, the vesicles, and adjacent tissues. This result is what will indicate, more assertively, the possible complete removal of cancer. If this does not occur fully, it will be necessary to continue the treatment with radiotherapy, since cancer cells may have contaminated other tissues, besides the prostate.

The new treatment would incur new risks, not to mention the continuation of uncertainties.

> The standard procedure for the cure of cancer involves the follow-up of a possible recurrence for an extended period of some years.

It is necessary to continue monitoring the PSA level periodically, since it will continue to be a marker for the presence of cancer cells, even without the prostate. Even so, with the excellent result of the pathology, I prefer to believe that everything is over, that I won.

When I think about the whole period, from the first suspicion until the outcome, I can watch two different movies.

The first one is of the happy ending, where everything seems wrapped in a beautiful gift package and seems to have passed quickly. After all, it was only two months and little until everything ended.

As I wrote earlier, suffering is much softer when it is memory than when feeling at each moment. Looking back is sweeter than actually being there.

In short, in this film, it seems that everything was not so wrong and that I see myself as if I were a third person, a character.

Much of this book has been noted down during my journey, when feelings were out in their moments, like fears, anguish, and uncertainties. If I watch the film of the journey from that point of view, trying to relive the feelings, then perception change, because I become aware of how difficult things were, and I will become the protagonist myself.

In this scenario, the film becomes a drama, at least for me it was.

Still, what matters is that this film also had a happy ending.

FINAL CONSIDER-ATIONS

I wrote some other books, although none of them even look like this in terms of reality and personal experience. Two of them were management books, focused on technology and business, and another one is short stories and chronicles, that is, fiction.

In all of them, including this one, in the end, I would like to achieve one main goal: to have contributed in some way to the readers, either by sharing information and knowledge or by helping them to be distracted (as was the case with stories and chronicles).

I hope that with this book, especially, I can help disseminate information and knowledge about prostate cancer, its diagnosis, and treatment. I expect to share reflections give useful suggestions that can help those who have to face a situation like this.

Every writer is appreciative of his or her readers, so this creates a paradoxical conflict for me. Some will read this book if they have prostate cancer, which is not a situation I would wish for anyone.

To be in the middle term, then, it should not be read by those who have cancer, but by those who want to be informed — informed about the importance of early diagnosis and the investigation and treatment.

If any reader wishes to make a comment or exchange information with me, or even point out an errata, please contact me through e-mail jst999@gmail.com.

Thank you very much for reading.

ABOUT THE AUTHOR

I am Juliano Statdlober, with a Bachelor's Degree in Economic Sciences and Postgraduate in IT Governance, an entrepreneur in the software business, a writer by hobby.

One (not so) beautiful day, at 53 years of age, I discovered to have prostate cancer.

I decided to write, first of all, to help me deal with the situation. Besides that, but not least important, I believe that the exposure of this kind of information is essential for the clarification and perhaps to help other people who go through this situation.

www.ingramcontent.com/pod-product-compliance
Lightning Source LLC
Chambersburg PA
CBHW051213250726
48655CB00006B/2387